Survival Lessons
from a Heart Attack

Survival Lessons from a Heart Attack

Angel N. Pagaduan

To order additional copies of this book, contact:
Xlibris Corporation
1-888-795-4274
www.Xlibris.com
Orders@Xlibris.com
63979

CONTENTS

DEDICATION

This book is dedicated to all readers who believe that—as a never-concretely-fathomable teaching of the Holy Scripture—"To God, everything is possible but to man, never!"

It is also dedicated to my wife, Marina, and to our children—Maria Theresa (Marisa), Susan, Adorico (Ricky) Jones, Marian, and Arlene, who all have remained steadfast adherents of a family-embraced Christian faith since sapling age.

Preface

An unexpected heart attack can occur without an otherwise beneficial warning signs, and any sudden death from it tends to often surprise us to incredulity—especially when the victim is a particularly known figure. But where zero fatality occurs, it hardly stirs as much fuss, and seldom—if ever—is how this factuality—as instead a matter of greater importance to discuss—engagingly talked about other than by surviving victims themselves—usually.

This complacency is traceable to science's confidence-boosting advances in the realm of the world's growing great wonders, which include debated though seemingly promising DNA/stem cell study findings. But still common sense teaches that in any surgically invasive application of medical technology to save endangered life, risk is ever present—even with employment of the best of modernity's discoveries.

Now, you as the reader may perhaps have heard stories of near-death experiences ending in either a tragic, permanent good-bye to loved ones for transition to an "everlasting life yonder above" or a recycled, "new life back here on earth." As a 76-year-old fairly healthy senior who unexpectedly suffered a sudden heart attack in 2007, I am lucky to have been blessed with the latter outcome. This is after I underwent a triple-bypass or open-chest, heart surgery in 2008 that inevitably bordered on only a 30%-margined chance of safety.

Because of the rarity of my surgical case compared to that of other heart patients with whom I had inter-changed medical experiences, "a sort of miracle and thus God's own will" is what I could only solely conclude out of all the healthcare help that I received for my greatly inspiriting recovery later.

So, next to God, for any healthcare guidance anyone may find worth gleaning from this book to reinvigorate his/her own wisdom of self-care for what earthly life appears to be fundamentally is for to mankind, to all those who had lent a hand in my "new lease on life" are due my endless thanks. There are many of them, and the most significantly responsible are mentioned in the pertinent pages of this book.

Indeed, whatever good readers may gain from the manifold, self-manifested lessons in this true episode of risk-studded life-and-death scenario is simply attributable to all who had been instrumental, directly or indirectly, in making its narration here possible—with me as a circumstantial vehicle.

In the chain of events surrounding my near-fatal but "luck-shielded" triple-bypass operation, those who have had variably a lot to do with my hurdling of it as the greatest danger I ever met in life are the following entities/persons (sequentially named according to source/category of healthcare dispensed in my favor):

Health Net Medicare:

Neena Batallones—Health insurance agent who enrolled me with Health Net

U.S./California Department of Health/Social Services (as a whole):

Hills Physician Medical Group (HPMG) # 857

Dr. Generoso P. Porciuncula—HPMG # 857 HMO physician who, under the routines of medical check-up, had well referred me for urgent cardiovascular evaluation

Dr. Gopala R. Kolluru—HPMG # 857 cardiologist who performed on me pre-surgical left-heart catheterization, coronary x-ray, and cardiac imaging, not mentioning other necessary subsequent cardiovascular/clinical routines

Washington Healthcare Hospital System (WHHS):

Dr. Kenneth T. Lee—WHHS cardiac surgeon who headed my triple-bypass operation

Dr. Dr. Sang H. Lee—WHHS cardiac surgeon who co-headed my heart surgery

Dr. Robert Hsu—WHHS physician who lent vital assistance throughout my case's major phase

Other WHHS healthcare teams comprising nurses, medical secretaries, respiratory and physical therapists, medical technicians, and cardiac rehabilitation workers

Post-Surgery Immediate Healthcare:

Terri Lane—PHCA case manager who took charge of home-visit/monitoring evaluation for me

Moral and Spiritual Support:

Rev. Seamus Farrar and Rev. Jun Manalo—St. Bede Catholic Church priests who lent moral as well as spiritual support thru inter-family friendship

Inter-family friends comprising Dr. and Mrs. Glecy Garcia, Beth Licad, Ed and Rose Manzano, Delia Alambat, Leny and Tom Ricafort, Bert and Gilda Wong—who shared part of their time visiting me in the hospital and at home or gifting me with well-wishing cards, including a snack stuff

Post-Operation Emergency Healthcare:

Dr. Jason Chu—Washington Township Medical Group, Inc. physician whose evaluation of my condition in convalescence resulted in his recommended "thoracentesis" in my favor

St. Rose Hospital

Dr. Jeremy Graff—St. Rose Hospital emergency physician who consequentially advised cardiovascular referral for ensuring normalcy of my recovery

Al Presto—St. Rose Hospital ER staff nurse who quite appreciably carried out all necessary clinical routines for me

Dr. Michael Maiman—St. Rose Hospital radiologist who performed "thoracentesis" on me, resulting in my great relief from breathing difficulty in my condition of heart failure

WHHS Cardiac Rehabilitation Center:

Ivar Blomquist, MS, ETT—Cardiac Rehab Exercise Therapist

Phyllis Fiscella, RN, CDE—Cardiac Rehab Clinician/Certified Diabetes Educator

Lani dela Rama, RN, MSN—Cardiac Rehab Clinician

Introduction

We all are not immune to heart attack, a health scourge dreaded by either sex as the most common cause of sudden death among people of all walks of life—rich or poor, famous or not—particularly in the U.S. Some victims felled down by it end up lucky survivors, but incidences of its occurrence with hardly any noticeable, presaging symptoms at times had often resulted in unexpected death—even in early or prime age, hence its unsettling stigma: indiscriminate "# 1 silent killer" almost anywhere.

Although devoid of a significant filial history of heart disease or any of its seen tributaries—diabetes, hypertension, obesity, etc., I happened—as a 76 year-old, fairly healthy senior—to fall victim to it, and only a triple-bypass heart surgery was to later save me.

This is after a "stent" was first installed in my heart four months earlier when one afternoon I just suddenly felt a bit dizzy, nauseated, and disoriented. My 911 call resulted in doctors' findings of (painless) "myocardial infarction"—with me fully conscious and normally breathing but only a little discomforted as thus described.

Urgent, remedial insertion into one of my chest arteries of a plastic, spring-like devise called "stent" to normalize blood flow in my heart immediately followed at the St. Rose Hospital, Hayward, California. I was hospitalized there on November 2, 2007, and released a day thereafter, or on the 4th.

But the following four months after my "stent" treatment saw me occasionally suffering again from momentary recurrences of chest pain (called angina) like before—and this went on for about a two-month period prior to what was to later emerge ultimately as my only savior: triple-bypass heart surgery. New blockages (formed by blood clots) were found in my heart; so, under a last-recourse but what to me then was a self-expected promise of modernity's life expectancy-prolonging technology, "Yes"—without any second thought—was what I perforce readily said to my cardiovascular doctor, following his advice of a triple bypass heart surgery for me.

A bleeding complication, however, rendered my surgical case to tether on a margin of safety with only a "30%-chance" for survival; it in fact alarmingly turned out as the "first and only one of its kind from more than a hundred" that was ever handled by my heart surgeon. With my hurdling of it nonetheless thus unsettlingly but fatefully exuding a rather miraculous tone, it was successfully performed at the Washington Hospital Healthcare System, Fremont, California, on April 11, 2008, under the auspices of Health Net Medicare, my insurance provider contracted under the auspices of the U.S. Department of Health.

It was during my ordeal of regaining post-operation consciousness that I experienced what I could only recall as an extremely stressful, agonizing moments of near-death impact. Foremost was that as I struggled to awaken myself from what palpably was just a fractional consciousness (out of anesthesia's subsiding effect), I felt as if I was enshrouded with a blanket of darkness where the only other thing contrastingly visible was a pair of light fronting my eyes. In form, it assumed the semblance of two dazzlingly luminous, sun-like figures displayed with an irregularly outlined circumference—one partly superimposed over the other with equal, virtually blinding brightness amidst total darkness.

In this scenario, I audibly sensed a nurse repeatedly calling my name to wake me up, but could only remain totally immobile and restrainedly incapable of reacting in any way. At the same time I felt seeing my surgeon who, although not fully recognizable because of the sight-blanking darkness fronting me, appeared silhouetted gesturing that I make a motion to raise my right forefinger in the way he demonstrated. This, after and by sheer persistence, I was at last able to do!

Then, following what seemed a quite palpable upsurge of relief in my throat after my surgeon had held me intently as if to let it happen, my senses just became fully resuscitated at the same time from what I could only recall as a sort of a hellish "stupor-paralyzed consciousness." With my consciousness thus fully restored from what simply seemed a near-death moments' tight clutches, I just felt able to normally talk again as usual, as well as respond to those around—quite a welcome relief indeed from the then extremely distressing physical weakness and seemingly invisible body shackle that for some time hindered my usual easy mobility.

As I sort of felt freed at last of the physically painless but summarily unbearable agony of it all, the foremost sense that just unfolded in my mind—right after being literally unburdened of the moment's darkness that earlier stressfully enshrouded me while motionlessly supine on bed—was the overwhelmingly inspiriting thought: "How great indeed is the omnipotence of God!" And this at the same time made me feel just profoundly grateful in silence—with the words of Christ (as I learned years ago from the Bible), "In God, everything is possible; in man, never," then just following in my mind.

These almost spontaneous and other purely spiritual matters of circumstantial relevance were then what practically obsessed me later with what I could only sense and feel as a way to a "new life" gloriously repaved for me. And as background, it is this unforgettable experience of rebirth—out of what simply was a brush with a near-death, agonizing ordeal—that led to this book.

In turn, this book affords what could be a veritably engrossing front-seat view of actual experiences from which fellow laymen could beneficially learn first-hand lessons on (particularly) how to avert, if not totally evade, an oft-fatal, surreptitious peril of human aging: unexpected, sudden heart attack from just nowhere. But, as is true of my case, etiological origin is the natural inevitability of arterial thickening—or "atherosclerosis"—as regrettably prodded then by my own utterly naïve attitude about a particularly fat-rich food that I have become complacently fond of.

For side lessons, it tells as well or in passing, among other pertinently informative matters of medical import, of risks always associated with carelessness in, or ignorance of, taken medications, prescribed or self-secured.

PART I

Pre-Attack Scenarios of Health-Related Issues

Wrong Belief about Heart Disease

Like most people, I had always held the notion since adolescence that heart disease, particularly "heart attack," is largely hereditary. Cases of families I personally know to typify this in a from-parent-to-children pattern added weight to this belief. And chiefly for this reason, I, as the oldest of a ten-member offspring progenitor-ed by parents whose immediate and even remote ancestors hardly had a significant trace of hereditary heart disease, have always harbored the thought that never would I ever be affected by cardiac trouble.

Thus, by this erroneous confidence plus an absolutely carefree attitude that made me remain carelessly undiscriminating for decades in the kinds of food I eat, I just stayed particularly fond of pork and beef. And—on almost regular, weekly basis—my favorite is what doctors would always surely caution their heart patients against: pork entrails cooked first with water and salt, then fried, in their own remnant lard-laden state, into a semi-crackling dish. "Chicharon bulaklak" is what it is called in Pilipino.

Aftermath of Food Misconception

My knack for pork intestine cracklings went on through the years particularly during my adulthood. Starting on my 60's, my eating of it increased to an almost weekly basis.

But this lasted only until after I reached 76, or on November 2, 2007. This arose portentously a necessity as a result then of what was to fatefully happen with me in the afternoon of that very same day: seeing myself just suddenly feeling, with hardly any expectation, a bit dizzy, nauseated, and disoriented. In short, I saw myself unexpectedly a victim of sudden heart attack—without what I had all along learned about years earlier as symptoms often preceding or accompanying it: chest pain and/or difficulty of breathing.

As I was to think to myself regretfully later (with nothing whatsoever held in my thoughts about the natural results of aging), I simply was wrong in my belief that what is a taboo kind of food to others who became victims of sudden heart attack would not adversely affect me.

But then, as what diagnostic routines—electrocardiogram, blood test, etc.—were to later establish, my cardiac attack proved to have been primarily caused by the narrowing of the interiors of my arteries, and this was said to be due to long-time plaque deposits on them as a natural (but not uncontrollable) consequence of aging.

Doctors medically call this "atherosclerosis," a health imperfection inevitably given rise to in the process of anyone's getting older.

But undoubtedly in my case, it was enhanced by the particular kind of fatty food I then had become very fond of as circumstantially the major, triggering cause of it all: "chicharon bulaklak!"

Sudden Onset of "Burning" Sensations of Pain in My Chest

Within and for about two months before my heart attack, I found myself just suddenly discomforted—and this is for the first time ever—by a sort of "burning" sensation that invariably felt like a mild, infernal-like but somehow bearable pain in the center area of my chest.

Lasting for about a couple of minutes every time it occurred, this kind of physical pain just suddenly came by once to three times a week, irrespective of whether I was at rest relaxing or otherwise, i.e., physically or mentally preoccupied.

Its occurrence was hardly predictable, with its characteristic, concomitant pain dissipating little by little afterwards. "Angina" is the medical term I was to later learn about that is used for it.

Sudden Onset of Irregular Heartbeat

As my angina grew oftener starting on about a week prior to my heart attack, with me holding on the speculation—not without some worry under the circumstance, of course—that I was perhaps only suffering from an ordinary indigestion-rooted heartburn, I just suddenly started experiencing a slightly palpable heartbeat irregularity.

But unlike my angina, its occurrence was seldom, and its palpability became particularly easy to sense whenever I prepared myself for sleep.

When my heart attack did occur, I just felt in my chest a momentary heartbeat irregularity for the last time while I was on bed, within a night of just about three days before the attack.

Other than this, there was nothing whatsoever that made me presciently feel as something significantly worrying enough for me to expect that what was an already brewed or perilously impending heart trouble was then about to actually get unleashed on me.

Long-Term Medications Preceding My Myocardial Infarction

For more than ten years already before I had my heart attack, I have been taking prescribed medications necessary for normalizing my high blood pressure, thyroid function, and uric acid level in my blood.

Atenolol (50 mg.) is the medication I take daily for my high blood pressure, which began to develop in the mid 1990's, or when I was nearing my mid 60's.

Levothroid (125 mcg.) is what I take every day as well for my low-performing thyroid gland, whose function was said to have been mal-affected by the cumulative effects of past and repeated X-ray-generated radiation. I began taking Levothroid more or less at the same time as I started with Atenolol. It is my doctors' advice that my Levothroid medication is a "must" throughout my lifetime.

And Allopurinol (500 mg.), which I take at also a dosage of one tablet a day, is a prescription intended as a preventive medication against attacks of gouty arthritis on my joints. But my taking of it on long-term basis is—and this was what my doctor had advised—for seeing ultimate dissipation of the lumpy uric acid-salt deposits on the joints of my feet and hands. To my own gladdening observations, my doctor's advice does go on actually taking place effectively—with my on-and-off gouty attacks rendered all but absolutely inexistent now.

A later long-term medication prescribed for me to lower my cholesterol when a routine test showed a high level of it in my blood is Simvastatin (80 mg.), taken once a day. I began taking it on about just a few months before my heart attack.

For many times, though, I often forgot taking it and this ranged from once to twice a week. When I had my heart attack, the first regretful thought I had was about this medication irregularity, which I had rather neglectfully concerned myself with at the beginning.

I thus could only endlessly blame myself later—thinking that my having otherwise taken Simvastatin even only as a neutralizing precaution—perhaps—against my fondness for fatty foods, which are rich in cholesterol, might have somehow slowed down my heart attack's occurrence, if not staved it off completely.

But whether or not I am right in harboring this thought remains a pure conjecture to this day, and only cardiac specialists perhaps could provide a right, enlightening answer.

Impelled Stoppage of Smoking

When I had my heart attack, I had about twenty years of smoking behind me. At an average cigarette consumption of 10-20 sticks a day that variedly included brands like Marlboro, Philip Morris, Chesterfield, Lucky Strike, and Camel, both filtered and not, I had once and for all quit the habit in the early 1990's. Chewing uncooked rice and drinking a lot of water whenever urge to smoke arose helped me quite consequentially in finally ridding off the habit.

This was following two successive acute respiratory infections that saw me hospitalized within a period of about a three-month interval between each confinement.

Antibiotic injections cured me of the infections—and precluded their recurrence as well. But my doctor had found me already about to develop the early stages of a lung disease called "emphysema," for which he perforce could only advise that I should stop smoking completely if I am to avoid the certitude of its aftermath of eventual fatal complications.

While I at last succeeded in quitting the habit after six successive but futile attempts earlier, each of which lasted only about three months at the most, I did not totally escape what I could only think of as its cumulatively resultant ill-effects: occasional respiratory discomforts characterized by wheezing, little coughing, and on-and-off mucous formation—particularly in cold months.

For relief and as a recommended palliative when necessary, I was advised to take Robitussin, an over-the-counter cough medication labeled as equally a good expectorant and cold decongestant. It has since proved effective for what it is, but my need for it has now become seldom.

Near Fatal Cold-Spurred "Bronchial Spasm"

Undoubtedly because of my previous years of smoking that eventually made me suffer from its after-effects in the way described above, I once experienced a sudden shortness of breathe that nearly saw me respire for the last time to death.

Prior to this nearly fatal incident, which took place upon my arrival at home from work one afternoon, I had a four-day-old severe cold that necessitated my taking of Robitussin to help ease the difficulty of my breathing, a malady that I then could only ascribe to the clogging of my nose with thick mucous. My discomfort with this respiratory trouble typified the kind that usually arises from a common but tight cold, and use of the Robitussin palliative recommended for me to use against it did have—as was the case in many occasions—some quite relieving effect.

But in the afternoon of about the fifth day of my cold discomfort, I just suddenly felt as if my lungs could not normally expand as usual for inhaling as I am ordinarily wont to do. In such condition, I had to laboriously gasp for air—with my lungs' capacity to suck it in (for normal respiration) just suddenly rendered all but totally zero.

Greatly alarmed, I felt impelled to call 911. On being asked how I find myself under the circumstance, I exactly described over the phone that "I just suddenly experienced difficulty in breathing," and that "my discomfort is not necessarily in my nose as is usually the case with a severe cold, but in my bronchial area—with my lungs seemingly incapacitated and unable to expand or contract."

When an ambulance arrived shortly thereafter, the attending paramedic immediately made me inhale—through my mouth and with use of a portable mist-exuding device—some kind of a gaseous medication which, to my great relief, just readily enabled me to breath normally again. This was done as an emergency step while I was in the ambulance, on the way to the hospital.

At the Kaiser Hospital in Hayward, California, diagnostic tests resulted in findings that I had a severe "bronchial spasm," preceded by symptoms of asthma and/or bronchitis—particularly with respect to wheezing and mucous formation in my bronchial structure.

"Albuterol" is the medication (dispensed from a mist-producing plastic inhaler) I was made to take and after a few hours of my stay in the hospital, I was released with advice to use the aerosol medicine only when I encounter again any instance of breathing difficulty.

It was a little over two years before my heart attack when I first had this kind of bronchial trouble, and to this day I have no idea whatsoever whether or not this malady is etiologically connectible to any kind of cardiovascular disorder. As it is, up to the present, I never had a "bronchial spasm" again since then.

Primordial Gouty Arthritis

The first time I suffered from an unexpected onset of this kind of arthritic, joint malady—which most people usually associate with humans' natural aging process—was more than thirty years back or before my heart attack in 2007. It (initially) occurred sometime in my mid 40's, and occasionally went on until put under control by my medication Allopurinol starting on the later 1980's, or after an elapse of some fifteen years (I was nearing the 6th decade of my age then).

Gout's most particularly unbearable, nerve-wrenching symptom as I actually experienced it twice up to three times a year is a seemingly gnawing, sharp pain on the joint of my right foot and toe. An attack usually stayed for one to two weeks, with the swelling and soreness affecting the skin and tissue area of my toe gradually dissipating as days went by.

So sensitive would my affected toe become whenever the malady sets in that even the slightest touch on it by what supposedly is a blanket's softness readily invites a sharply acute, unbearable pain. And to walk on any instance of the malady's attack period, which would just suddenly occur on any month of the year, turns into an extremely agonizing moment because of searing pain generated every time any pressure of walking weighs down on my affected foot.

Another characteristic symptom of gout is the formation of lumps on the joints of my fingers, in both right and left hands. Doctors consensually attribute this to accumulation of uric acid salts deposited on my fingers' joints.

Whatever direct cause is actually responsible for my gout, I like to think that I inherited a susceptibility to it from my mother, who, until her 90's (she lived up to 93 after a triple-bypass heart surgery when she was 84) showed telltale indications of it in the form of gouty arthritic lumps on her fingers.

But over the years the sizes of the uric acid lumps on my fingers gradually diminished. My sustained Allopurinol medication, which did a lot of good in preventing recurrences of what once were my periodical bouts with painful onsets of the malady, appears to be significantly instrumental.

Tophus Surgery

Due to the growth on my right toe of a tophus about half the size of a golf ball over the years that made my wearing of shoes painful, I was compelled to have it excised out by orthopedic surgery.

The operation was done at the Oakland Highland Hospital in 1987. A local anesthesia was used that made my entire lower half body numb. This rendered the operation totally painless, with me fully conscious.

But the operation did not mean prevention of recurrences of my gouty attacks. A new tophus, in fact, gradually developed again but this time it was on my left toe. It did not grow to as big a size as my first tophus, though, thereby sparing me of the need for another orthopedic surgery.

Stomach-Bleeding Aftermath of "Endocine" Medication

"Endocine" is the name of a drug prescribed beginning in the late 1980's for my use every time I had a gouty arthritis attack. It proved effective in controlling arthritic swelling and pain but in the long run resulted in a nearly fatal intestinal bleeding that only an emergency operation had effectively remedied. This was sometime past the early 1990's or when I already had totally stopped smoking.

Occasional use of the drug over some years made me realize that the mere drinking of milk prior to medication (milk was advised by my attending doctor at the time for me to drink first in case I had not taken any previous meal) contributed to the brewing and eventual onset of my stomach bleeding problem.

But it was actually aspirin (as and for self-medication) that exacerbated my intestinal bleeding when I was compelled to substitute it for "Endocine" after I happened one night to get short of the latter's supply at home.

This took place coincidentally while I had a gouty attack on my left foot's toe. Because of my growing weakness and continuous excretion of black stools that resulted shortly thereafter, I was treated at the Emergency Clinic of the St. Rose Hospital some time in the early 1990's. Intestinal operation followed by regular "Zantac" medication eventually cured me of my stomach bleeding ailment. And to this day never have I again found myself affected by it—about twenty years from the time I first fell victim to it.

Occasional "Colchicine" Medication

In place of "Endocine" or any other for-pain-and-swelling drug for my recurrent gout, my Medicare doctor had preferred prescribing "Colchicine," which I then would take only when the extent of my gouty attack so warrants from the standpoint of its severity and/or of my capacity for pain tolerance.

Despite its after-effect of causing me to become prone to loose bowel movements once maximum dosage is reached, it proved quite relieving of gout's main discomforting symptom: joint pain and swelling.

But my use of it lasted only ephemerally, and this is chiefly because of the fact that my Allupurinol medication had in the long run appeared quite just as effective in forestalling the ailment's recurrences, thereby rendering my use of "Colchicine" all but totally dispensable for quite some time now.

As it is, I have not been taking it since the mid 1990's, or starting with my mid 60's.

Recovery from Major Ailments without Prescribed Medications

Malaria, dysentery, and typhoid are three kinds of diseases commonly known to have a predisposition to sure cure/control only through medications with proven drugs.

But during my early teen's when the World War II (historically) gave rise to a dearth of medicines in conquered countries, I, as one of many who got sick one after the other of these maladies within about a three-year period, happened to be lucky in overcoming all of them without any prescribed medications.

As recollections were to later make me think why, I could only think—for an answer—that perhaps my natural immunity or DNA-based body defenses might have somehow accounted for my having overcome and survived the three otherwise serious ailments.

True, some home-prepared palliatives—like sweet vinegar-wet cloth application on the forehead in times of malarial and/or typhoid fever, drinking of a severely bitter concoction from a (boiled) herb called "darita" (said to be a raw source of quinine for malaria), etc.—seemingly did have some alleviating effect whenever taken by me.

But, as I was to later recall, this effect could have (attributively) resulted more perhaps from a psychological rather than a really curative standpoint.

For what simply could a valid, scientifically conclusive explanation be made for one's getting cured of such otherwise sure-killer diseases as just aforesaid, if not the likelihood that genes must have somehow played what actually might have been their inherent role under the circumstance.

Penicillin Allergy

In my late teens, I got sick of a skin-mouth ailment that was etiologically ascribed by a doctor to poor diet, and Vitamin C deficiency was said to be the root cause in my case.

Initially, the ailment affected my mouth, and my skin followed in subsequent periods after several recurrences in my mouth. It occurred once to twice yearly—and whenever in my mouth, it manifested itself in the form of localized ulcers on my tongue or on my lips.

Its occurrence on my skin assumed the form of slightly elevated rash-like appearances that tended to heal in the middle section while at the same time peripherally expanding until complete healing time that spanned a period of more or less a month.

My eating of certain kinds of sea food like shrimp, salted fish, or crab tended to aggravate my discomfort with the ailment, and only by avoiding them while affected and by eating more of fruits seemed to hasten my trouble's disappearance.

As an attempt to (speculatively) forestall recurrences, I took almost blindly every brand of widely advertised over-the-counter multi-vitamin tablets.

Also, in my consultations with different doctors, they saw it permissible for me to have penicillin injections as well. This began on the ailment's second occurrence, and it continued with every recurrence of it. At that time penicillin was the most recently marketed # 1 antibiotic popularly known to be quite effective against many kinds of infections, and its prescription for me was purportedly to see me cured once and for all.

But cumulative results eventually proved contrary to expectations. Where penicillin shots appeared somehow helpful in ridding off my mouth-skin ailment every time it reoccurred, the question of why the injections fell short of their supposed efficacy against any recurrence remained an unresolved enigma.

For as was to later surface to an inescapable transparency, it eventually turned out that my repeated use of the vaunted antibiotic seemed to have at last reached a so-called "point of diminishing returns!"

And this is best describable only by way of the fact that I just found myself most overwhelmingly perturbed for the first time by abrupt skin eruptions that were to later get correctly diagnosed as my allergic reaction to penicillin over-usage.

What served to solidly support this is the fact that beginning with the first and after just about 24 hours following a dermatologist's prescribed treatment with an oral medication called (and sounded) "Methycortylone," which I took simultaneously with an intravenous Vitamin C injection, I got readily relieved and resultantly "cured once and for all" of my mouth-skin ailment. This was in my mid 20's, and I never had seen myself bothered by it again since then.

PART II

Onset of Attack & Related Happenings

Backdrop and Moment of Attack

Since birth to adulthood, I simply had not known of any (guiding) reason for me to think—even remotely—that I would ever encounter a heart attack. As I had earlier mentioned in this book's introduction, non-existence of any significant kind of heart disease in my ancestral lineage sort of counted to me a circumstantially plausible explanation.

And if my occasional, pre-attack moments of "burning" sensations of pain in my chest should otherwise have portended to me a telltale sign of an impending heart disaster then, whatever significance this was supposed to presciently convey amounted to anything but meaningful. Mindlessness ended up regrettably with the misjudgment that such pain is just the result of an indigestion-caused heartburn. In other words, naivety-nourished complacency additionally contributed to seeing my self-stumble into a careless, nearly life-ending aftermath.

And then it just happened all of a sudden! I had just arrived at home from work on the afternoon of November 2, 2007, when, after lowering my head a little in the process of gurgling to wash my mouth on a sink, I just suddenly felt a bit dizzy upon straightening up my body.

Under the circumstance, I felt for a moment as if my sense of balance—i.e., of seeing things in front of me—was not normal. Illustratively, what I felt was typical of or akin to how one feels after turning around his head many times or in a way that he is not wont to do. Mild and somewhat dizzying disorientation aptly sounds to be the right description for this.

As it was my very first experience to see myself thus affected, with me feeling somewhat instinctively urged at that same instant to vomit out of my stomach rather than out of my esophagus (as if for automatic relief out of the moment's nauseating discomfort), I perforce had wisely decided to call 911.

I then could hardly find it right under the circumstance to drive myself to the hospital, fearing that my (prompting) discomfort, even if just slight but nonetheless actually disabling, could jeopardize traffic safety into detrimental aftermath to all and sundry.

911 Call's Administered First Aid

It took just about ten minutes for an ambulance to arrive, in response to my 911 call. I then had described in advance exactly what and how was I feeling when I was asked pertinent questions relative to my call. This, I believed, helped greatly in enabling the two paramedics, who were to later attend to me at home, in knowing exactly beforehand what they needed to do for the emergency.

And the very first thing they did upon arriving and seeing me seated while I was in the act of throwing out but actually nothing whatsoever to vomit off at all was to gauge my blood pressure and temperature.

"Two hundred plus (systolic) over 100 plus (diastolic), you have a very high blood pressure!" was what the lead paramedic could only exclaim after reading the measurements he had taken of me.

He right there and then took out some aspirin tablets for me to ingest, after also exclaiming "You have just a heart attack!"

When I told him—from a reminisced past allergic medical reaction—that the aspirin might result in a bleeding of my stomach, he could only assure that it was the emergency moment's extremely necessary, sole remedy for me. And he added the explanation that there could be some other possible, protective medicines which doctors could prescribe for me later or as need arises.

The succeeding moment saw me carried on a portable bed unto the ambulance waiting outside my house. Once inside the vehicle, I was made to put on its fixture's hanging respiration-aiding device for emergency oxygen supply.

But all through the duration of my emergency situation the only discomfort I felt was just my being a bit disoriented—and not without some perturbing nervousness, of course, despite my having not experienced at all even so much as an iota of such commonly known and usually ominous heart attack-related discomfort as shortness or difficulty of breathing.

And the fact that even in my being already of age 76 at the time it was only a disorienting slight nausea that bothered me and not other kinds of discomfort like chest pain, shortness of breath, or loss of consciousness (to which most other heart attack victims usually succumb) served to rather indicate nothing short of a "strong heart."

"Stent" Insertion into My Heart's Artery

After examining and diagnosing my case routinely by stethoscope, X-ray, blood test, electronic scanning, and electrocardiogram, attending doctors had found out that I was afflicted with a cardiovascular disorder. Three of my heart arteries were said to be involved in plaque formation over the years. I was to later learn that this is due primarily to high cholesterol-food constituting my diet, other ordinary consequences of human aging put aside. The plaque formations in my arteries are said to have stemmed from calcium and cholesterol deposits.

Preparatory to their application of needed remedy, the doctors had decided that a "stent" was what appeared to be the best cure for me under the circumstance.

Made up of a plastic spring-like device, it was inserted into one of my heart's arteries—necessarily to restore normal cardiac functioning for my entire circulatory system, and thus let a steady supply of oxygen and nutrients conducted to where vital in the body.

For the process, a sort of hole was made in my groin area, and through this hole was passed something that made the operation possible towards a painless conclusion and curative relief for my heart condition.

During this non-open chest operation, I was asked to describe what and how I felt as a sort of thin (plastic or rubber?) tubing was procedurally manipulated into my heart arteries (I understood it to be the three thickly "plaque-ed" ones).

Compliantly, I answered as exactly as what and how I actually felt as each manipulation proceeded, concomitantly with a nurse's scan-aided questioning. And all that I felt was practically the same kind of "burning" sensation of pain as what occurred in the center of my chest area every time my angina arose months before.

Other than this sort of "burning" sensation, there was no pain whatsoever that occurred palpably to my senses as my attending heart specialist went about his chores of stent-treatment for my heart ailment.

As far as I could recall, I could only think that I sort of underwent also an "angioplasty" during or as a procedural part of the treatment. I received no general aesthesia whatsoever, and I was made to remain fully conscious all through the operation.

Purportedly—and true to what I was to later actually experience, my "stent" had made it possible for blood flow to again normally take place in my heart.

As I was made to understand later, blood flow into my heart was rendered all but totally stopped during my "cardiac infarction," thereby mal-affecting supply of (blood-conveyed) nutrients particularly oxygen to my brain—hence my proneness to feeling dizzy in my situation, with the tendency to vomit or "through out" being a concomitant effect.

"Oh, it seems it's been all a miracle!" was then what I could only exclaim to all those around after my "stent" treatment was completed, and this was when one nurse had more or less casually remarked at the time that I was lucky in my particular case: I was fully "conscious when brought in (to the hospital's Emergency Room), unlike others who are otherwise."

If this is actually how I exactly felt about the operation on me, it is because I unexpectedly just found myself greatly relieved—immediately after the treatment—of all the discomforts that my heart attack had then just suddenly—and rather ominously, too—afflicted me with earlier: slight dizziness, disorientation, and tendency to vomit!

In short, my "stent" treatment had succored me out of an otherwise fatal cardiovascular disorder. It proved quite effective circumstantially as the only means of seeing my usual state of health restored—with a non-sanguinary efficacy achieved in a way that could only make me ultimately feel later as if nothing at all but a virtual "miracle" had happened to me.

Post-Hospitalization Precautions

Post-"stenting" routine observations saw me released from hospitalization just after only about 48 hours, or right on the third (from the first) day, of my confinement.

For my post-emergency protection, the medication Flavix (75 mg.), at a dosage of one tablet a day, was added to my list of needed (prescribed) medications. It is intended for thinning blood or as a protection from occurrences of arterial blood clots—which are known to predispose cardiovascular patients to heart attack.

As extra protection, I was also later given pamphlets seen useful in adopting a new lifestyle observant of proper dieting, exercise, and avoidance of ill-health promoting habits including smoking and immoderate drinking—which happened to be inapplicable to me as one not so habituated.

And most important of all, I was released with a tickler slip for making a "must" appointment at the end of the following three months with a cardiologist for a tread mill test—understandably for sure assessment of my recently administered heart stent's post-operation status or ultimate efficacy.

Temporariness of Feelings of "As If Nothing Had Happened with Me"

All through the entire three-month period following my heart-"stent" treatment, I had not felt anything wrong whatsoever with my health to make myself worry endlessly about. My health condition stayed just as normal as usual—no bodily pains whatsoever or instances of breathlessness or dizziness, a characteristic condition usually known to typify common symptoms of heart ailment, among others.

But this markedly changed starting on the fourth month following my treatment. And the underlying purpose of my "stent" specialist's own standing advice then for me not to fail having a check-up of my condition in a "must" medical appointment for a treadmill test at least three months after the treatment simply proved indispensably important; it was to subsequently serve as a more reliable medical basis for a relatively better way out of the same original problem that I was to eventually re-experience.

As I had herein described earlier, I again found myself just suddenly suffering from a mild burning-like sensations of pain or angina as before. At the same time, I also began getting easily fatigued, with my feelings of tiredness and concomitant weakness occurring more quickly every time I walked longer distances. This was to such extent that I had to stop walking in order to rest and rebuild my energy, as well as let my angina disappear.

Result of "Must" Treadmill Test

Thus, when I did get a cardiologist's appointment (through the intercession of my HM0 or Health Management Organization physician, Dr. Generoso P. Porcuincula, of 1251 W. Tennyson Rd., Ste 1, Hayward, CA 94544) for the urgency of my treadmill test, I could only be doubly grateful for the findings thereof.

Conducted by Dr. Gopala R. Kolluru, M.D., of the Hill Physicians Group of Hayward, CA, the test indicated that I still am afflicted basically with cardiovascular disease, notwithstanding my "stent" treatment.

And the fact that I tended to tire and gasp for air quickly in performing the test's timed and electronically monitored requisite of strenuous walking yielded definitive results of nothing less than a portentously resurgent heart trouble for me.

By this, further tests were then consequentially seen quite urgently in order. But they were to be in the form this time of a series of "heart catheterization," "coronary X-ray," and "cardiac imaging." These tests' results altogether turned out conclusively unfavorable but in a way quite vitally providential.

"Three of your heart arteries have all become clogged, leaving only a bypass operation as immediate solution—better than, and instead of, your waiting until you suffer another heart attack" was what could only be quipped in full context to me by Dr. Gopala R. Kolluru, my cardiologist. Aware of my situation ("that is prone to a more serious heart attack"—as I could only then think to myself under the circumstance), I right there and then I could only agree, in response.

My Open-Chest Operation—and Its Compounded Risk

After undergoing all routine and other necessary preparations following prior arrangements and approval by the HNM (Health Net Medicare), I was operated on for my heart disease's (actually) second administration of treatment—but this time under the category of a "triple-bypass" or open-chest surgery.

It was done at the Washington Hospital Healthcare System on April 11, 2008. My cardiac surgeon is Dr. Kenneth T. Lee, whose accompanying anesthesiologist is Dr. Sung H. Lee. They were assisted by a team of medical staff comprising nurses, technicians, etc., with an assistant physician leading in the person of Dr. Robert Hsu.

Due then to my blood thinning medication Flavix as necessitated after my "stent" treatment since some five months earlier—actually to help safeguard against blood clotting on certain unpredictable conditions in my case, I consequently became prone to risky bleeding of any cause. I thus could only conduct myself with nothing but sheer faith of reawakened fervor under the circumstance—solely speculating but strongly hoping that counter measures vis-à-vis this risk are well within a margin of tenability for my circulatory normalcy, positive chances for my post-surgery prognosis similarly not put aside in my mind.

"My days ahead are all within only God's will" was what then I could only completely resign myself to and think of for whatever was actually in store for me.

Ordinarily, among most patients undergoing such kind of major open-chest surgery as mine, it has become a common notion that chances for one's success in pulling through all risks involved have technologically improved through the years—reportedly and to my own knowledge—up to nearly 100% in most cases.

But in my case, it proved otherwise. As I was to later know, my chances for (surgical) survival converged on only a low 30%-level. This was said to be primarily rooted to the fact that it took a relatively longer time for my surgical bleeding to stop, with blood transfusion entailing up to four bottles of clinically supplied blood during my operation.

As my cardiac surgeon could then only exclaim in whole sense shortly after I regained consciousness from my surgery, "You bled, we had to take you to the operating table twice, and your case turned out to be the first and only one of the kind I had ever handled, out of more than a hundred!"

To me, nothing in retrospection bespeaks of a more risky surgical scenario of near-death reality than what my cardiac surgeon had described indeed! And I find it simply worthwhile to here picture all the actualities of it, trusting that each relevant fact as it actually happened would concretely speak for itself.

Surgery Case's Unsettling Indicators of Serious Complications

As a matter of common knowledge, there is hardly any doubt that complications associated with major heart operations ordinarily arise and are not impervious to fatal consequences in some cases—with weak body constitution of patients, mistakes, etc. proving equally contributory risk factors.

But what arose in my case happened to be more than particularly alarming to me.

And what rather sounds with an uncanny factuality out of what my cardiac surgeon had said of my particular case is simply true.

Aside from my Flavix medication's inevitably compounded (but nonetheless necessary) risk (of profuse bleeding) as was then typified to nearly my own doom on the operating table, I was to thereafter still tread for a time on a miscellany of some other post-surgery potholes of perturbing complications, disregarding their own respective alarming dangers.

Sleeplessness and Poor Appetite

Almost throughout my three-month period of convalescence, I remained greatly bothered by sleeplessness and poor appetite, which by themselves are not easy but stressful enough to cope with as health erosive problems. The mental and physical pressures their depressive effects on me simply assumed an extent of such rigorously debilitating hardship that anyone so affected just would feel loathed to even

imagining to have again the (circumstantial) kind of heart surgery
I had. No pain whatsoever had discomfortingly bothered me, but
feeling now and then with low energy as I experienced it throughout
my convalescence was simply all but bearable.

Extreme Thirst

Another most unforgettable effect of my surgery's complications is
my having quite uncomfortably experienced—and this was the first I
ever had in all my life—an extremely acute yearning for water during
my stay in the hospital's Intensive Care Unit, where I was attended
to for three days first before I was transferred to the ordinary care
room.

The intensity of want in my mouth for water grew into such degree
that—practically under simultaneous spells of extremely nerve-racking
mental and physical discomforts—it drove me into ceaseless moaning
for even just a gulp of cool water—for even so much as the slightest
(imaginable) fleeting moments of thirst-quenching relief from it.

"You cannot yet drink water as much as usual because it would
be bad for your condition, but here's ice (some pieces in a cup) you
can have and melt in your mouth to sooth yourself with for the time
being!" was what my attending nurse could only advise me to do under
the circumstance.

For three days, this was how my routine went for moistening—at the
most—the seemingly bottomless pit of thirst amidst my overwhelming
anguish, and I just could not but think, in my recollections, that sheer
strength of will, among other possible factors, somehow contributed
to my having overcome the really quite hard situation I found myself
in.

Unexpected Loose Bowel Movement

Still another suffering I underwent was my being rendered just
suddenly unable to control my bowel movement. Unexpectedly

occurring on about the second day of intensive care given me, it was only ephemeral, with no recurrence on any other day. But my discomfiting experience under the circumstance was simply embarrassing! A whole piece of linen got inevitably stained with a smelly watery waste to such extent that it necessarily had to be entirely rid off and replaced in my bed.

What unexpectedly happened to me this way was just so censurably discomfiting indeed, and it was only the attending nurse's palpable condescending compassion for the gravity of my condition—as she herself had understandably sensed—that dispelled my feelings of self-blame.

Sensations of Body Heaviness and Onset of Congestive Heart Failure

A further, markedly unsettling anguish I grappled with was that on about the third day after my surgery, I started feeling as if I had become abruptly heavy in my whole body. This was to such extent that I simply found it all but easy to move about as usual on my bed.

As I could then only conclude to myself upon gradually noticing my puffed-up body particularly down to my feet, the cause was edema, a condition given rise to by my body's mal-affected capacity to rid off unnecessary liquid (supposedly) through my kidney's normal functioning.

With my whole body appearing like it has somewhat bloated, plus my markedly sudden physical weakness and proneness to hard, short-interval breathing, **"congestive heart failure,"** was what arose to manifest itself as the most alarming, singular after-effect of my surgery. "Oh, Lord, I hope not yet but still roomy for me on my days ahead" was how my thoughts could only run in silence every time I cast my eyes on my boated body!

The situation I found myself in simply kept me worried so deeply that I just could not but remain dispiritingly uncertain of what is to actually happen with me as my convalescence went on. If there is anything that steadfastly kept me optimistically looking forward, it was sheer faith in what I could only look up to and value as God Almighty's transcendental power "over and for everyone"—as I then could only think to myself.

And then under the circumstance there, too, was what simply remained to be quite material in the scene of it all: a constantly alert and regular medical monitoring, which then had consummated into seeing me afforded every circumstantially warranted dispensation of care and cure.

In the end, I could only feel profoundly grateful for emerging freed of all the dangers that confronted me in the entire duration of my post-surgery convalescence in the hospital, where I had to stay for about week, and then at home for about a three-month period thereafter.

Morale-Building Effects of Caregivers and Callers' Well-Wishing Visits

The fact that all those who attended to me during my surgery and hospitalization—doctors, nurses, therapists, etc.—had done so with a really soothing, contagious graciousness proved by itself to be more than enough for all the optimism that morally strengthened me with, towards my full recovery. The general aura of kindness they had manifested as mirrored in their smiles and benign, "howdy" greetings is such that I just felt everything is going on fine with me.

And what proved significantly material as well in sustaining my morale—specially during my stay in the hospital's critical care unit—were the comforting moments of loved ones' almost daily visits to me. Their self-manifested, worried facial expressions as palpably engendered by how I must have haggardly looked to them in my overall physical condition mutely stirred feelings of "all is not well" about myself under the circumstance. But this nonetheless greatly helped in keeping my spirits impervious to on-and-off moments of pessimism that cyclically filled my mind as one in grips with the particularly risky heart surgery that I just had gone through.

Even long-distance, well-wishing calls, which all appreciably conveyed to me a special personal concern for my particular case, more or less also injected an uplifting dose of morale nourishment.

The making of any kind of body movement on bed in the situation like mine while under standing precautionary instructions restrictive of certain physical exertions tends to always invite careful, second thinking before doing so. In my case, this paled against what simply sounded as sort of a counterpart harbinger of spirit-lifting social nicety that is expressed across hundreds of miles away, just for ensuring my well-being as one with an unexpected life-threatening ordeal in his early twilight years.

Indeed, hearing the voices of loved ones from across a continent even as it entailed not-easy-to-make physical bodily movements is simply like feeling exhilarated out of a popularly adulated singer's voice even as it meant standing strenuously long amid the inconvenient jostling of a throng.

Post-Hospitalization Happenings

When about a week after my surgery on April 11, 2008, I was released from the hospital, the first thought I had was "Oh, at last, I am already far from danger!" With great relief, this was how sort of silently elated I was about my condition under the circumstance. And enhancing my gladness about it is that—in keeping then with my cardiac surgeon's advice—I did manage to have a daily physical exercise by continuous walking for 20-25 minutes without any untoward bodily sensations. And the fact that I also continued to receive post-hospitalization home-visit monitoring/nursing care 2-3 times a week made all the more assuring for me that I really was well on the way to an already-danger-free recovery.

But on about the 5th week of my home convalescence, a markedly worrisome change in my condition just suddenly emerged. Congestive heart failure unexpectedly resurged—with it concomitantly manifested by edema on my (puffed-up) feet and by my sudden proneness to short, hard breathing, as well as tiring easily even on slight physical exertion.

I thus felt constrained to seek immediate medical attention at the nearest hospital to my home. After less than a day's stay in the St Rose Hospital's Emergency Room where I underwent tests on blood chemistry and electrocardiography including chest X-ray, I was advised to immediately see my cardiologist for needed remedial steps towards improving my condition. By Dr. Gopala R. Kolluru's advice and arrangements in conjunction with the recommendations of St. Rose Hospital's ER Physician Dr. Jeremy Graff who attended to me quite graciously with the assistance of his equally gracious Staff Nurse Al Presto, readjustments were made in my medications. Also, "thoracentesis" as warranted by my having developed "pleural effusion" was scheduled to be administered to me.

Under to-each-medical-specialist's-own-authoritative expertise, all of the different steps taken to improve my condition proved simply nothing less than so much to thank for. Not only did I eventually overcome with great relief my congestive heart failure and its characteristic symptoms of discomforting proneness to easy tiring and short-interval breathing but also able to resume normally my usual daily chores as before.

Resumption of "Lassix" or Furosemide (20 mg) Medication

When my congestive heart failure first occurred—and this was on about the second day following my triple bypass surgery, it was a prescribed medication called "Lassix" or Furosemide (20 mg) that proved almost singularly instrumental in curing me of my operation's really worrisome # 1 complication. I took it along with Potassium Chlorate, supposedly to neutralize whatever adverse effect Lassix may cause while I am on with it.

But my having stopped taking of both medications when I had consumed all of what were prescribed unexpectedly just gave rise to my congestive heart failure's resurgence—and this took place on about the 5th week of my post-hospitalization recuperation at home.

Thus, it is only after resuming (until necessary) my Lassix and Potassium Chlorate medications—as then urgently advised by St. Rose Hospital's Dr. Jeremy Graff on about mid May 2008—that I got eventually relieved of all of such discomforting symptoms of a resurged congestive heart failure as edema, body weakness, easy tiring, and on-and-off shortness or difficulty of breathing. The original prescriptions for both medications were made by Dr. Robert Hsu and the renewed ones, by Dr. Gopala R. Kolluru.

"Thoracentesis" as a Key to My Further Relief from Congestive Heart Failure

For a corroborative attention on my surgery's complications—and thus ultimately for my further relief, my attending cardiologist, Dr. Gopala R. Kolluru, had referred me to Dr. Jason Chu of the Washington Township Medical Group, Inc., where the necessary facilities and expertise suited my case. There, I underwent breathing treatment; also, I was given written recommendations for a "thoracentesis," a vitally supplemental treatment that I was to receive on May 21, 2008, at the St. Rose Hospital. Administered by the hospital's radiologist, Dr. Michael Maiman, it consisted in the utilization of a syringe for drawing out excess fluid from my left lung, with an ultrasound electronic device facilitating the process. Prior to its execution, I had to suspend, by doctor's advice, my "Flavix" medication for three days first, to preclude possible profuse bleeding during the puncturing of my left lung, through my back, with a syringe's needle for fluid removal.

When it was done, I felt as if everything about my health condition has suddenly returned to a greatly satisfying, mind-easing normalcy. I felt my breathing to be no longer as laborious as it rather was prior to the treatment, and my tendency to get tired or lose energy easily after just some efforts of walking had ebbed away. And luckily for me under my situation, the temporary three-day stoppage of my Flavix medication did not cause any adverse effect on my circulatory flow.

Other Health Restoring Measures during My Recuperation

Within the remaining few days following my "thoracentesis" treatment, RN Terri Lane, a PHCA nursing case manager assigned to render home-visit care for me, happened to be still on task as such.

Her periodical visitations to check and monitor the progress of my convalescence at home procedurally saw inter-clinical phone-communicated arrangements that resulted in immediate alterations in the array of medications I had been taking in conjunction with my bypass surgery. Two medications covered for this are "Metropolol" and "Amiodarone HCL"—which were both dropped off my list of prescribed medications at the time. As I was made to understand relative to this change, the purpose of dropping off of both medications was to help bring my lowered blood pressure up to a normal range—and result did eventually see attainment of this goal.

Before my taking of either or both, I had told my attending cardiologist that there were times when I occasionally experienced what I felt as rather my pulse's irregularity on my wrist. His findings about this with supplemental use of an electrocardiogram in the course of my pre-scheduled post-surgery appointments in his clinic accounted for his prescription for both medicines.

There are other medications that got procedurally dropped off what was prescribed for me to take during my post-surgery convalescence—"Potassium CL 20 Meq," "Amlodipine Besylate," and "Furosemide 20 Mg" tablet.

One kind of drug prescribed for me to take whenever I experience any instance of pain is called "Hydrocodone-Apap 5-500," but my having never found myself affected by any kind of pain at all throughout my recovery had made its use dispensable.

If the miscellany of medications prescribed for a heart surgery patient can be a window to the gravity of his/her medical case, then the wide variety of my medications as such all through the course of my recuperation self-reflects affirmatively my own case's seriousness.

Involuntary Thoughts about My Surgical Case

Undoubtedly, the greatly satisfying consequence of all the inputs of care given for my relatively alarming heart surgery has had a lot to do primarily with the latest technological wonders of medicine as a science. All those entrusted with its practice in my case, directly or indirectly, are undeniably instrumental as well.

But what keeps on predominantly self-unfolding or looming in my mind over and above this is rather the involuntary, irrepressible thought that God's ever unfathomable omnipotence is the most instrumental of it all.

My surgical case happens to be fated with a post-operation prognosis of somewhat grave, multi-faceted complications, and who else but God could be the only (never-fathomable) entity that must have willed my hurdling of all of the risks associated with it, inherently or otherwise! And if all my attending doctors' expertise, not to mention others concerned and modernity's myriad technological advances, have collectively been responsible as well, still it is to me a part of only God's will that they all were providentially employed as such under the circumstance.

Relative to this, I then consequentially just could not help but think, too, that in my high-risk or only "30%-safe" surgical case, a teaching of the Bible attributed to Christ, "In God, everything is possible but in man, never," had by itself seemingly found and manifested a coincidentally phenomenal occurrence of a quite relevantly hard-to-deny attestation.

And the fact that I am already well past middle age or an elderly of 76 bordering on life's twilight years (initially?) at such period is in itself an extra risk is particularly something that rather all the more pertinently sits well with these three firmly (self-) believed possibilities—as since then irrepressibly etched in my mind: 1) Inherent result of genetic factors; 2) Benefits of modernity's technological advancements plus medical expertise; 3) and God's own will—as ultimately the determinant architect of it all.

That there are those who would hardly similarly hold and believe in this trio of thoughts is understandable, given the fact that it is one of the ordinary characteristic qualities of human nature. But for anyone to intently entertain the seemingly rationale but never-possible idea that it is only after the real "how-aspect" of life's earthly beginnings is discovered could be proven the reality of God's existence as an all powerful Creator (primordially) responsible for the Big Bang itself is simply like one trying to equal what is all about within the very domain of God's power only. As most would agree, any analytical imagination, if not common sense, is prone to always make it clear that this could never be possible in any way. This is self-explained right in and by the fact that if it is otherwise, then whoever could make it possible would simply appear to be no less than "another existence" (or a replicate?) of humanity's supposedly one and only true God!

Curious Coincidence between Publication of Written Book and My Prognosis

When I had my bypass operation, it happened that a book on proven but limitedly known ways of above-par learning among students that I had written (from cumulative 30-year exposure to practically every nature of all grade-level classroom situations) was undergoing publication (by Xlibris.com).

The book's pre-publication elicitation of others' richly positive assessment of its palpably fadeless utilitarian worth as a (surely) handy referential guide towards A-1 schooling anywhere carries such weight that I just then could not but tell my cardiac surgeon, after his briefings with me on my operation: "You know, doctor, far from impertinence but I happen to now have a hitherto untold, stimuli-rich guidebook for boosting student performance but with certitude to see print and use only under positive chances for my surgery."

As to actually then turn out thereafter, despite my cardiac surgery's "only 30%-chance for survival," I did manage to pull through it saved—and the book, titled *How to Get "A" Grades in School*—with the sub-caption "A 10-Tickler Formula for Smart Learning," is now in print for general readership.

Purely coincidental or not, wishful thinking (or what not?), this simply is something that makes me feel unabashedly inclined towards the belief that it is all a will of God.

Why or how this could ever solidly gain concrete plausibility, if not solidly unassailable validity, is somehow analyzable out of several coincidental but factually relevant instances.

Most relevantly significant is the fact that the book happens to parallel in a way the Bible—not for purposes or in the domain of religion but education—with the following expected as sure outcomes: 1) Upped learning performance to achievement levels proportionate to the extent at which students would follow the book; 2) Concomitant character enrichment via its stimuli-rich, inspirational real-life illustrations vis-a-vis every ilk of schooling misconduct including truancy, academic disconnection, and acts of extraneous or covert nature; and 3) Perpetual usability as a pragmatic means/resource by which parents—even under once-in-a-while progress check amid their busy hours—could vicariously reinforce desired efficacies supposedly of their own home counseling for their children's schooling.

In this regard, it is pertinent and worthy to mention that the book happens to integrally touch on, in its topic, "Let Yourself Delve into Education's Vital Role in Life," which is discussed on its page 28, the creationism-tinged sense of the excerpt from it that reads entirely thus:

"We all need education in life, a one-way journey we undertake through time for the pursuit of activities that make for our general well-being for as long as our mind, body, and soul—as well as health allows. Since no one can ever validly gainsay or deny this because it is universally felt and seen—a truth deriving in turn credence only from the kind and strength of faith existent in us, most humans including even the most famous of scientists themselves could not but hold and believe that life is God-given and education is not. For this reason, we all need to acquire education for enriching our mind with knowledge and thence go on with and enjoy life assured of a worthy future: enhanced usefulness to ourselves, families, and the society we live in—even to all humanity itself!"

PART III

Post-Convalescence Developments

Heart Rehabilitation Program

As part of the Washington Hospital Healthcare System's established procedures for the benefit of its post-bypass surgery patients, I was included in a group of them that underwent a two-month cardiac rehabilitation program. For the batch I was listed with following a recommendation from my cardiologist, Dr. Gopala R. Kolluru, I participated in it 2-3 days a week, from July to September, 2008. The class I attended was regularly held at the WHHS Cardiac Rehabilitation Center, 2500 Mowry Avenue, Fremont, California.

The program consisted in participants' undergoing of physical activities (including breathing exercise) for an hour on each day of their respective schedule of class attendance. Ultimately for the purpose of helping strengthen the heart, all participating patients, under choices of their own for the kind of physical exercise that is made possible with an assortment of electronically controlled aerobic facilities—treadmill, stationary bicycle, etc.—performed physical exertion routines supervised and consummated with monitored blood pressure, pulse rate, and other health-related data.

The obvious cardiac-rehabilitating benefits the program provides are so highly appreciated by participants themselves that they all are practically in unison enthusiastically performing all of the different forms of physical exercises every participant likes to engage in, in a hall spaced optimally for accommodating up to 20 persons at the same time.

"I just am glad that I am in this program . . . it's been more than 10 years now since my heart surgery, and I just feel quite fine," was what one jolly senior participant had casually quipped to me when I first attended the July-September 2008 batch of participants in the program.

Insofar as I am concerned, the program's particular value to me is that I simply had learned quite a lot better and in a much more comprehensive way about the really great importance of regular physical activeness as simply the most natural means of healthily maintaining the physical capacity of everyone's heart to desired levels of normalcy.

Implementation of the program is made possible through the healthcare services of three to four nurses/physical therapists.

Readjustments in Medications

Within a part of my post-convalescence period of recovery, or starting on about the 5th month after I had my surgery on April 11, 2008, a series of follow-up assessments on my general state of health pointed to the need for some changes in my medications. Based on blood tests and routine physical-medical examinations conducted separately but coordinately by my cardiologist, Dr. Gopala R. Kolluru, and by my HMO physician, Dr. Generoso P. Porciuncula, my to-date (as of May 16, 2009) list of medications is as follows:

Name of Medication	Dosage	Times/Day	Particulars
Allopurinol (for gouty arthritis)	500 mg	1	-
Amlopidine(for hypertension/angina)	5 mcg	1	Started 03/09
Aspirin (for heart attack/stroke)	81 mg	1	-
Atenolol (for hypertension)	50 mg	2	Dosage upped

Carfate (anti-ulcer complication)	16M/10Ml	3	2 teaspoonfuls
Ferrous Sulfate (anti-anemia)	325 mg	2	-
Flavix (for heart attack/stroke)	75 mg	1	-
Folic Acid	1 mg	1	-
Levothyroxine	125 mcg	Mon, Tue, Wed- 2 Tue, Thurs, Sat, Sun- 1	-
Simvastatin (for cholesterol control)	80 mg	1	Restored in replacement of Pravastatin Sodium 40 mg

Carotid Doppler Test

One year after my surgery, or on April 2,009, at my cardiologist's behest, I underwent a Carotid Doppler test in his clinic. Its result indicated a ("small") blockage, but it was evaluated not of a magnitude posing such level of danger as to suggest the need for even so much as any form of curative surgery. All that is then concluded for me to understand and accordingly observe is simply maintenance of my ongoing adopted post-surgery, modified living style, continuance of all my medications (as listed above) plus careful, high cholesterol-free diet and engagement in adequate exercise, the everlasting importance of sufficient sleep and fresh air not mentioned.

If a carotid artery electronic examination was seen necessary for me, it is because of atherosclerosis' possibility of causing me to suffer also from a stroke—similarly an etiologically leading origin of a sudden onset of death, if not permanent disability, as a result of plaque buildup. As it is said, the buildup of plaque along the walls of diseased arteries—a condition assessable via ultrasound technology applied on a carotid—can restrict blood flow to the brain or break off and become logged in a blood vessel, causing a stroke. It is thus that I perforce have to maintain caring for myself via the list of medications I have been taking since the onset of my heart condition and then after my surgery.

Self-Assessment of Current General State of Health

Thanks to the quality of all of the healthcare attention lent me as a senior now nearing 78 who had an almost fatal (30%-safe) bypass surgery a year ago after a stent-treated heart attack four months earlier, I just feel myself currently in a generally good condition.

My appetite has returned (from the time I was operated on) to a satisfying level of normalcy, just as my sleep. I have not so far felt any kind of pain in any part of my body nor in my head. Also, my respiratory system has remained generally normal, with my wheezing no longer as loudly bothersome and frequent as before I had my surgery. Further, my almost weekly blood pressure self-check up at home or in a pharmacy since my full recovery stays showing results describable as anything but alarming—and this parallels my doctors' own findings in my periodical clinical check-up. To sum it up all, I just feel myself to be doing well—physically and mentally.

oooooOOOOOooooo